RELAX YOUR MIND

COMPANION WORKBOOK

A GUIDE TO LEARN MEDITATION TECHNIQUES TO RELIEVE STRESS AND QUIET A BUSY MIND

THOMAS CALABRIS

Check out our website at:

www.EliminateStressNow.com

Relax Your Mind Workbook
Publisher: Inner Vitality Systems, LLC.
Website: www.EliminateStressNow.com
ISBN: 978-1-951382-00-1

Disclaimer

The Information presented in this publication is intended as an educational resource and is not intended as a substitute for proper medical advice. All readers are encouraged to seek proper professional and medical advice when needed. This book is not for anyone that has medical mental conditions. Do not read this book and seek proper medical treatment if you have a serious mental illness.

The author and publisher of this material are not responsible in any manner whatsoever for any action or injury which may occur by reading or following the instruction in this document. The author cannot be held responsible for any personal or commercial damage caused by misinterpretation of the information or improper use of the information.

No patent liability is assumed with respect to the use of the information contained herein. Although every precaution has been taken in the preparation of this book, the publisher and author assume no responsibility for errors or omissions.

TABLE OF CONTENTS

Quotes From "Relax Your Mind"

"All it takes for you to be in the "here and now" or the present moment is for you to make a choice. Make a choice to live in the present moment."

"So when we talk about relaxing the mind, we mean to let go of all the mental chatter and to quiet the mind."

"Visualization is one of the most powerful techniques for retraining your mind."

"Another way to root yourself in the present moment is to sit quietly and focus on your breathing."

GETTING STARTED

I hope that you have had a chance to read the *"Relax Your Mind"* book or at least have started to read it. It will give you the background and understanding of the meditation techniques mentioned in this companion workbook.

To get the most out of this workbook, I recommend completing each section in the order presented. You will benefit the most by taking action daily and working on the sections in this workbook. Be consistent and patient. Have fun with it.

Consistent practice is required to relax and reprogram your mind. However, don't try to force any outcomes. Everyone gains the benefits in their own time. Trust in yourself and just keep practicing.

I recommend that you write your experiences down. You can use the spaces provided throughout this workbook. Longer-term, you should consider investing in a journal. A journal allows you to focus and reflect on your experiences along your journey to *"Relax Your Mind."* During trying times, when you have doubts, it is important to look back at your progress and successes to keep you motivated and moving forward.

Also, after you learn the meditation techniques, I recommend creating a weekly action plan, as shown later in this workbook. It will help you to keep track of your progress and experiences. You can also keep your action plans in your journal.

Also, your action plan will help you to consistently increase your conscious awareness and work through what is stressing you out, causing your fears and how you react (unconsciously or consciously) to fearful or stressful events. Daily practice will help you make progress towards accomplishing your desired outcome on your way to *"Relax Your Mind."*

I encourage you to have an open mind as you go through the material in both the "Relax Your Mind" book, as well as this workbook. While the ideas and techniques may seem different than what you have experienced in the past, I urge you to find out for yourself how powerful they are by committing to practice them daily.

Now let's get started by identifying the root-causes of your stress.

WHAT IS STRESSING YOU OUT?

If you want to relax your mind, then you need to be honest with yourself. What is stressing you out? Remember that fear is the root cause of all stress. Answer the following question to get to the cause of your stress.

Question: What fears are the root cause of your stress?

Write down your answer:

_____

_____

_____

_____

_____

_____

_____

_____

_____

_____

_____

_____

_____

_____

_____

Choose To Live In the "Here and Now"

We experience life in the present moment, the *"here and now."* However, sometimes our stress negatively programs our subconscious mind by worrying about the past or the future. To completely relax our minds, we must become aware of our negative actions (programs) to our stress triggers. We do this through *"silent witnessing."*

It is through our actions that we gain experience, so it is now time to practice *"silent witnessing."* Take note of the times you are thinking about the past and the future. Also, notice your fear and stress triggers. What makes you angry, stressed, anxious or fearful? Write them down. Repeat this daily.

Past and Future Thoughts:

_____

_____

_____

_____

_____

_____

_____

_____

_____

_____

Fear and Stress Triggers:

FREE YOURSELF WITH FORGIVENESS

Sometimes in order to live in the present moment, we must do some work to let go of the past. This may include forgiving. Holding a grudge can consume a lot of your emotional energy, which keeps your attention in the past. It also keeps you from living in the present moment and it keeps you from living a life of peace and gratitude.

You may need to forgive someone in your past that has done something bad to you. That doesn't mean you have to accept their actions, but you need to forgive them in your heart to truly let them go. You don't necessarily need to forgive them in person. You can just forgive them in your mind and heart. Then you can move on with your life and live free in the present moment.

You may also feel you need to be forgiven for things you have done to others. Do you regret saying something that hurt a close friend? Did you pick an argument with your spouse just to get attention? Whatever it is that is keeping you stuck in the past, you need to resolve it and move on. Now is always a good time to apologize and say you are sorry for your actions to those you have hurt. Yes, this is difficult work, but it is more difficult to live years with regret. And it keeps you from the deep healing needed to find inner peace.

You may also need to forgive yourself for making a bad decision, or letting your health go, or whatever it is you blame yourself for. As the saying goes, "We are often our own worst critics." We are sometimes harder on ourselves than others. No one is perfect. We don't have to be perfect to live our best life. Are you a perfectionist, needing to get everything just right?

Now take inventory of everyone in your life, past or present, that has done something to you, that has caused you to hold a grudge, anger, jealousy, frustration, disappointment, sadness, or any other negative emotion that keeps you stuck in the past. Write down the person's name and what they did to hurt you. After that, make a statement to forgive them for their actions and wish them well. Yes, wish them well even if you don't feel like it and even if you can't say it to them in person. Remember, this is for you, not for them. Then make a statement that you are now free to live in the present moment. For example, *"John stole money from my home, and we are no longer friends. I forgive John and hope he finds whatever is missing in his life and I wish him well. I am free from John's actions and can now live in the present moment."*

Forgiveness inventory of others that hurt me:

_____

_____

_____

_____

_____

_____

_____

_____

_____

_____

_____

_____

_____

_____
_____
_____
_____
_____
_____
_____

Now take inventory of the things that you did that have hurt others. Include actions that you have not been forgiven for like saying something mean to a loved one, borrowing something without permission, cheating on your boyfriend or girlfriend, and others. Be honest with yourself. This may be the most difficult task in this workbook, but it is worth the price for relaxing your mind and finding inner peace. Write down the person's name and what you did to hurt them. After that, make a statement that you will apologize to the person and ask for forgiveness. At your earliest convenience, take action to visit the person and apologize. For example, _"I hurt Jane by lying to her and then she found out. I will ask Jane's forgiveness because our friendship is too important."_

Forgiveness inventory for people that I hurt:

_____
_____
_____
_____
_____
_____
_____
_____

_____

_____

_____

_____

_____

_____

_____

_____

_____

_____

_____

_____

_____

_____

_____

_____

_____

_____

_____

Now take inventory of the things that you did that weigh on your mind. Include actions that you have not forgiven yourself for things like overeating regularly, lying to your spouse, not paying the bills on time, getting fired, and others. Be honest with yourself. You need to understand all of the deep-seated emotions that are keeping you stuck in the past. Write down what you did to hurt yourself. After that, make a statement to forgive yourself and wish yourself well. Then make a statement that you are now free to live in the present moment. For example, _"I fell for an email scam, and it cost me a lot of money. I now forgive myself for this mistake. I am now free to let this go and to live in the present moment."_

Forgiveness inventory for myself:

_____

_____

_____

_____

_____

_____

_____

_____

_____

_____

_____

_____

_____

_____

_____

_____

_____

_____

_____

_____

_____

_____

GRATITUDE IN YOUR HEART

Gratitude is one of the keys to living in the present moment. It is difficult to be stressed when you feel gratitude. What are you thankful for? Write down five new things you are grateful for every day.

1. _____

_____

_____

2. _____

_____

_____

3. _____

_____

_____

4. _____

_____

_____

5. _____

_____

_____

POSITIVE THOUGHTS

Positive conscious thoughts are key to focusing the mind. They are also important for retraining and eliminating negative subconscious programming. By focusing on positive thoughts, we create new neural pathways for these positive thoughts. And since we are not focusing on the negative thoughts, the neural pathways for the negative thoughts are not enhanced and will diminish over time. Here are some examples of positive affirmations to get you started.

1. I am calm, peaceful, and relaxed in this moment.

2. I am worthy and I am attracting abundance into my life.

3. I am healthy and I love my body.

4. I am courageous in all that I do.

5. I am forgiving and compassionate towards others.

6. I am aware of the choices that I make in every moment.

7. I believe in my body's ability to heal.

8. I can silence my mind whenever I choose to.

9. I choose positive thoughts about myself and others.

Now, create a positive affirmation that addresses your fears or stress. You may borrow from one of these examples, you can change one to fit your situation, or you can come up with something different. Be specific and creative.

Write your positive affirmation:

_____

_____

_____

_____

_____

In a comfortable position, quietly repeat your affirmation for at least five minutes. Now write down your experience. How did you feel? Was it easy or difficult? Be honest. Repeat this practice daily.

My experience was:

_____

_____

_____

_____

_____

_____

_____

_____

_____

_____

Take A Deep Breath

Breathing is a fundamental process of life. It energizes and relaxes the body at the same time. Begin a daily practice of abdominal breathing. Find a quiet place where you won't be interrupted. Turn off your cell-phone and other devices.

Sit down in a comfortable position. It is best to keep your spine straight, but not tense. Close your eyes and relax. Be in the present moment, the *"Here and Now."* Do abdominal breathing for two to five minutes to start. Remember the keys to abdominal breathing are **slow, long, thin, even, and soft**.

After your practice, write down your experience. How did you feel? What did you notice?

My experience was:

_____
_____
_____
_____
_____
_____
_____
_____
_____

_____

_____

_____

_____

_____

_____

_____

_____

_____

_____

_____

_____

_____

_____

_____

_____

_____

_____

_____

_____

_____

_____

_____

Practice abdominal breathing daily to get the most benefits. Schedule time to practice and make it part of your daily life.

Retrain Your Mind

Retraining your mind means to change negative unconscious thinking into positive thinking. This means you need to become aware of your negative thoughts before you can change them. Once you are aware that you are doing negative thinking on a regular basis, then it will be time to get to the root cause of this negativity. It is always fear.

What are the fears that are driving your negativity, worry, and anxiety? You can't eliminate your fears if you aren't aware of them.

Write down the fears that are driving your negativity, worry, and/or anxiety. These are likely the same that you identified previously in the "What is Stressing You Out" section. Be honest with yourself.

My fears are:

_____

_____

_____

_____

_____

_____

_____

_____

_____

_____

_____

_____

_____

_____

_____

_____

_____

_____

_____

_____

_____

For each fear, write down a positive way to deal with your fear.

_____

_____

_____

_____

_____

_____

_____

_____

_____

_____

_____

_____

THE POWER OF VISUALIZATION

Visualization is one of the most powerful techniques for relaxing your mind. Your mind can't tell the difference between an actual experience and an experience that was visualized. Visualization can help you to calm your mind and transform your life.

It is important to realize that "feeling" the experience you are visualizing is very important. Feeling allows your whole body to experience the visualization, not just your brain. Remember that if your visualizations are done correctly, your brain won't be able to tell the difference between an imagined or visualized event and the actual event.

Now let's practice. Find a quiet place where you won't be interrupted. Sit in a comfortable position and close your eyes. Don't lay down or you may fall asleep. Take a deep abdominal breath and let it go.

Visualize yourself in a situation that is calming and relaxing. Try to imagine all the feelings, sites, sounds, smells, and tastes. Involve as many of your five senses as possible.

For example, maybe you visualize yourself taking a peaceful walk in the park. Feel the warmth of the sun on your skin. Feel the cool breeze on your face. See the ducks swimming in the pond. Put a smile on your face. Sip on your favorite drink as you walk around and observe nature.

Continue to visualize in this way for five minutes or more. To conclude your practice, express gratitude for this time and your experience. Now write down what you experienced during your visualization. Did you feel like you were there? Did you feel calm and relaxed?

My experience was:

_____

_____

_____

_____

_____

_____

_____

_____

_____

_____

_____

_____

_____

_____

_____

_____

_____

_____

_____

_____

_____

Practice visualization daily to retrain your brain to experience calm and relaxation. Be creative and be patient. Have fun with it.

GET SOME FRESH AIR IN NATURE

Take some time from your daily activities to go outside and get some fresh air. Find a place that you can walk in nature. We are sometimes so busy that we forget about the beauty outside our doors. Walking in nature is a great way to relax and enjoy being in the present moment.

Schedule time to walk in nature. Do abdominal breathing as you are walking. Put a smile on your face. Be in the present moment and notice the things around you. What do you see? What do you hear? What do you feel? After your walk, write down your experience. Was it easy to be in the present moment during your walk? Write down anything that comes to mind about your experience.

My experience in nature was:

_____

_____

_____

_____

_____

_____

_____

_____

_____

_____

_____

THE POWER OF A SMILE

One powerful way to change your mood is to put a smile on your face. When you are in a good mood, you automatically smile. And since you have practiced this your entire life, you have already programmed your mind and body to automatically produce the chemicals necessary to feel good. Yes, it goes both ways. You can put a smile on your face when you are not in a good mood, and it will cause your mind to signal the body to produce the feel-good hormones. This is why we always put a smile on our face when preparing for meditation.

You can also visualize yourself smiling while you are accomplishing your desired outcome. Your smile will add another positive dimension to your visualization that will anchor it with feel-good hormones.

Here are some additional ways to use your smile during your visualizations. If you are upset or angry with someone, you can visualize yourself forgiving the person and giving them a loving smile. You can visualize it even if you can't do it in person.

If you have a pain in some part of your body, you can visualize the area healing and smile into the area and imagine the pain dissipating.

If you have difficulties speaking in public, you can imagine yourself telling an opening joke to break the ice and see the faces of the audience smiling and laughing.

See how powerful the smile is when used with meditation and visualization. Be open and creative. You will be amazed at the results of your practice.

Now it is time to practice visualizing with a smile. Sit in a comfortable position with good posture and close your eyes. Put a smile on your face. Visualize a situation that you want to achieve. See yourself accomplishing your desired outcome with a smile. How does it look, feel, taste, sound, and smell?

Once you have completed your visualization, write down your experience. Be honest.

My experience was:

_____

_____

_____

_____

_____

_____

_____

_____

_____

_____

_____

_____

_____

Ten Minute Relaxation Meditation

Daily meditation practice is a great way to relax and retrain your mind. I recommend that you add it to your daily routine, just like brushing your teeth. Before practicing, take some time to set your intention. What is the desired outcome you would like to achieve? This is your intention. You might want to be calm during a stressful situation. Or, you might want to have more positive thoughts. It could be to feel more joyful. Be positive, creative, and specific.

My desired outcome is:

_____

_____

_____

_____

_____

_____

_____

_____

_____

_____

Now come up with a simple positive affirmation that represents your desired outcome. Keep it positive. For example, I am calm, peaceful, and relaxed. Or, I am calm at work when I present at meetings. Or, I am calm and can easily go to sleep.

My positive affirmation is:

_____

_____

_____

_____

_____

_____

_____

_____

_____

_____

_____

_____

_____

_____

_____

_____

_____

_____

_____

It is now time to practice the simple ten-minute relaxation meditation that was explained in the book. The *"Ten Minute Relaxation Meditation Checklist"* has been reproduced for your convenience on the next page. Follow the checklist and start now.

TEN MINUTE RELAXATION MEDITATION CHECKLIST

Preparation

1. Find a quiet place to practice.

2. Sit up in a chair with your back straight.
   Feet flat on the floor.

3. Fold hands on your lap or put palms down on
   your thighs.

4. Close your eyes, take a deep breath, and let it out.

5. Put a smile on your face.

6. Set your intention for the meditation.

Meditation

1. Repeat your affirmation (1 minute)

2. Be in the "Here and Now", silent witnessing
   (1-2 minutes)

3. Abdominal Breathing (2 minutes)

4. Visualize your desired outcome (2 minutes)

5. Relax Your Body (2 minutes)

6. Finish your meditation with gratitude
   (1 minute or less)

Once you have completed the meditation for at least ten minutes, write down your experience. How did you feel? Was it easy or challenging? Be honest. Were you able to visualize your desired outcome? If you weren't able to visualize your desired outcome, try to understand why. Please know that you are worthy of achieving your desired outcome. Keep practicing, and you will get better at visualizing over time. Also, write down what you are grateful for.

My meditation experience was:

_____

_____

_____

_____

_____

_____

_____

_____

_____

_____

_____

_____

_____

_____

_____

_____

_____

_____

_____
_____
_____
_____
_____
_____
_____
_____
_____
_____
_____
_____
_____

I am grateful for:

_____
_____
_____
_____
_____
_____
_____
_____
_____
_____

KEYS TO A SUCCESSFUL MEDITATION PRACTICE

I hope you have practiced the individual meditation techniques and the ten-minute relaxation meditation, as described in the book and this workbook, at least once. Here's a list of key points to consider to have a successful daily meditation practice.

1. Practice daily. If you don't have time to practice the entire meditation, then just take one technique and practice it for a few minutes or longer. If you really want to learn how to relax your mind, then you need to make a choice and practice as much as possible daily.

2. You don't need to be perfect. Your meditation practice does not need to be perfect to get the benefits. Doing it imperfectly is better than thinking about doing it perfectly.

3. Choose to have more relaxation in your life. It is our choices that determine the quality of our lives.

4. Identify and let go of any fears that are occupying your mind. Once your fears are identified, you can write down positive actions to mitigate them. You can also use visualization to see yourself handling the situation gracefully in spite of your fears.

5. Know that you have the capacity inside you to retrain your mind. Remember that the brain is not hard-wired as we had been told. Neuroplasticity means that we can change the wiring of the neurons in our

brains. We should be even more excited to know that we can change our genes to improve our health and mind with our thoughts.

6. Create and repeat your positive affirmation daily until you have achieved your desired outcome. Then create a new positive affirmation for a new outcome. Rinse and repeat.

7. Invite a friend to join your meditation practice. They will enjoy the benefits, and they will keep you motivated.

8. Be positive. Have positive self-talk regularly.

9. *"Silent Witnessing"* works, but you need to put in the time and be patient. Everyone reprograms their mind at their own rate.

10. Live in the present moment, the *"Here and Now"*, even if it seems painful or unpleasant. If you try to avoid the pain of the present moment by numbing or escaping, you will negatively program your subconscious mind and you will make it difficult to make conscious choices in the future.

11. Live in a state of gratitude. Acknowledge what you are grateful for on a daily basis.

WORD SEARCH MINDFULNESS PRACTICE

It is important to remember to have fun along your journey to *"Relax Your Mind."* I have included two word search puzzles to give you a short break from your practice.

Actually, word search puzzles are the perfect tools for being mindful in the present moment. They are also great for focusing your mind. Focus your attention on the puzzle. Notice each letter as you search for each word. Don't entertain thoughts that are not related to finding the word you are searching for. If you find your mind wandering, just return your thoughts to your word search.

Any activity can be a mindfulness practice. When you are washing the dishes, just wash the dishes. Don't allow your mind to wander to thoughts of the past or the future. When you are taking out the trash, focus your attention on only taking out the trash. Be present as you take the trash out. It may seem obvious, but without being conscious of what you are doing, your subconscious programming will take over and it will control your thoughts.

So take your time and have fun as you search for the words in each puzzle. It is okay if you need a break mid-way through the puzzle. Enjoy.

Word Search 1

```
Y J X G K O S T R Q V Y D Y P U U D S H N
C C C Z S V S B Q B F R L C X X Q R R J P
J O H R O N O W K J A C S N G V R I S R D
K J A J N O O A N Y T Z Y L S R V D E N H
C E U V Z I E D P O S I T I V E G S I B J
F B R Q P T S N N O I T A T I D E M Y H X
O W Q U R A I I J B F T Z B F N R S C F E
R O W Y T X L M B A F D A W T U D E A L F
G N I H T A E R B L A N I M O D B A J M X
I D B K F L N U A E D Y O Y R A L E F L I
V N N F K E T O S L D M S J R I M L Y S H
E A B W J R W Y T P E U E T B L F D W O I
N E W R H I I N V N C O T V D Y B F C Q W
E R O B P C T I T O R M N I W P V R A T E
S E G Z Z J N A F U T U R E T R C V X N U
S H C O W E E R M K B P T O D A H K T I Z
W W O I S R S T F N W N O E V C R X T R U
G N L C O R S E E R F S S E R T S G X O S
O C X W M H R R G N P D C J U I J X S X N
O W G H S M C U S U B C O N S C I O U S D
Q N C F H T H E R W V X L M C E N W X Z V
```

Stress Free	Here and Now	Focus Your Mind	Present Moment
Meditation	Abdominal Breathing	Daily Practice	Forgiveness
Silent Witness	Retrain Your Mind	Subconscious	Positive
Relaxation	Return to Nature	Choice	Affirmation
Relax Your Mind	Gratitude	Fears	Future

Word Search 2

```
F J F E I L E R S S E R T S S E I R F A B Z
Z V I S U A L I Z A T I O N V S A E C L K X
J P I N O J U D G M E N T S J S C L J K J Y
L E M O C T U O D E R I S E D E T A M Y V E
F A T P C M L J Y E N I T J P N I X K K Q F
O C D S P E R O N C X Z H M G E O Y X X S Y
R E U E Y R Y N D H L J G U T R N O S L F F
G F C R E K W G E K V G U K U A P U U Q S S
I U L N S P M J J L Y O O S J W L R X P D F
V L S O A K B Z C X V K H B H A A B G J N R
E E C I T C A R P T N E T S I S N O C A I D
N O I T A T I D E M S S E N L U F D N I M I
E U X A V M M G E A Y M V X F O O Y R O R M
S I T X G L R E H P T B I C A I E L G P U N
S D G A U A N B S I P H T L E C O N D T O C
W K Q L T H F Y S J F H I M E S J H S I Y U
Q U I E T T H E M I N D S N N N H Z T W X E
M X F R W W M C N C H I O G G O D N S Y A K
Y U W E J B M Y M T Q G P J A C E G F E L U
L E C T S E G U N O A S H Y D T H W H Q E Z
V O L R H S A J A W A L K I N T H E P A R K
H N U L P P D V V A K M A I C T B H C Z P U
```

Stress Relief	Mindfulness Meditation	Relax Your Mind	Quiet the Mind
Visualization	Positive Thoughts	Relaxation Response	Consistent Practice
Grateful	Deep Breathing	Peaceful	Desired Outcome
Intention	Action Plan	Forgiveness	Conscious Awareness
Walk in the Park	Smile	Relax Your Body	No Judgments

PRESENT MOMENT MANDALA COLORING

Another great way to practice being in the present moment is by focusing your mind on coloring a mandala pattern. A mandala is a geometric symbol or pattern that has been used in Asian art for thousands of years for teaching, focusing the mind and relaxation. Mandalas are typically circular patterns that have been depicted as lotus flowers, wheels, trees, and jewels to name a few. [1] Coloring a mandala allows you to focus on the present moment on the intricate details of the pattern. Let go of the past and future. Be present and allow inner peace to fill your mind and body.

You will need colored pencils, crayons, or other coloring media to get started. It is very inexpensive considering the benefits that you will experience. If you choose to use colored markers or other wet media, like watercolor paints, please place a piece of cardboard between the page you are coloring and the other side to prevent bleeding through to adjacent pages. Note that the opposite side of the page will only contain an inspiring quote so that any information in this workbook will not be affected by bleed through. You will find three different mandalas for your enjoyment. Put a smile on your face, relax, and enjoy the calm.

References:

1. *"What is a Mandala? History, Symbolism, and Uses"*, Invaluable.com. Web Retrieved September 27, 2019 from https://www.invaluable.com/blog/what-is-a-mandala/.

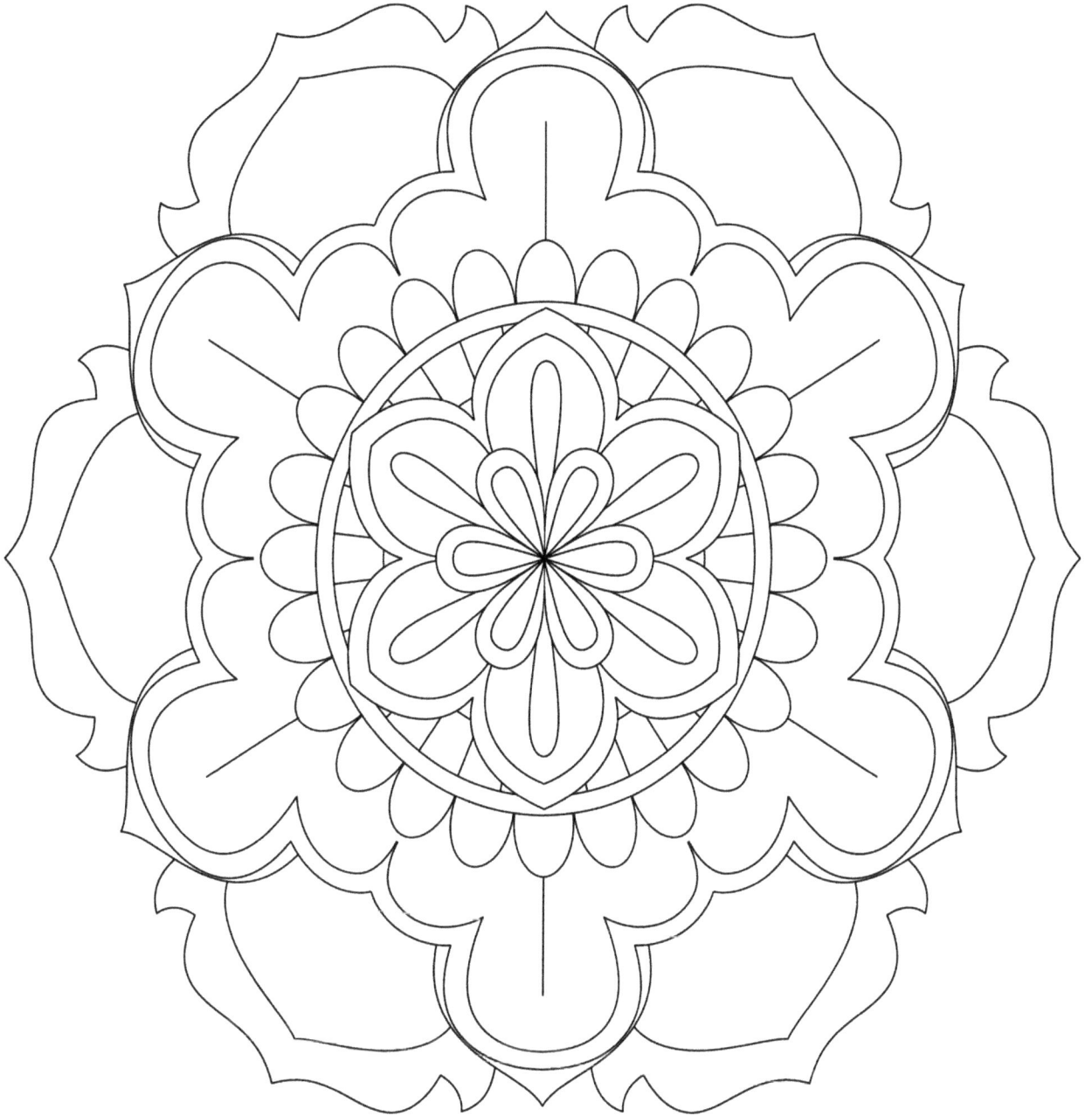

"You don't have to see the whole staircase, just take the first step."

– Martin Luther King Jr.

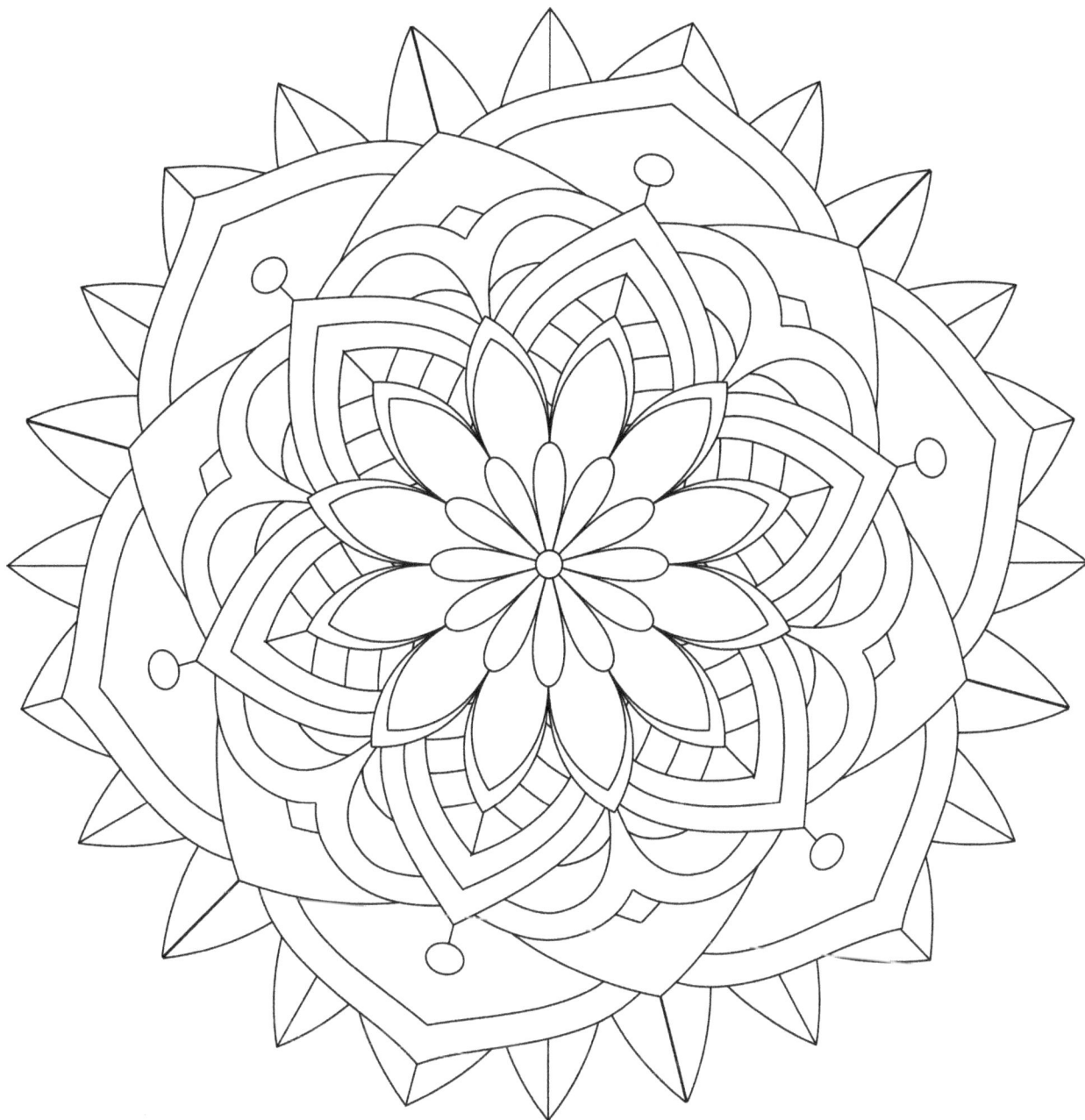

"If you truly love nature, you will find beauty everywhere."

– Vincent Van Gogh

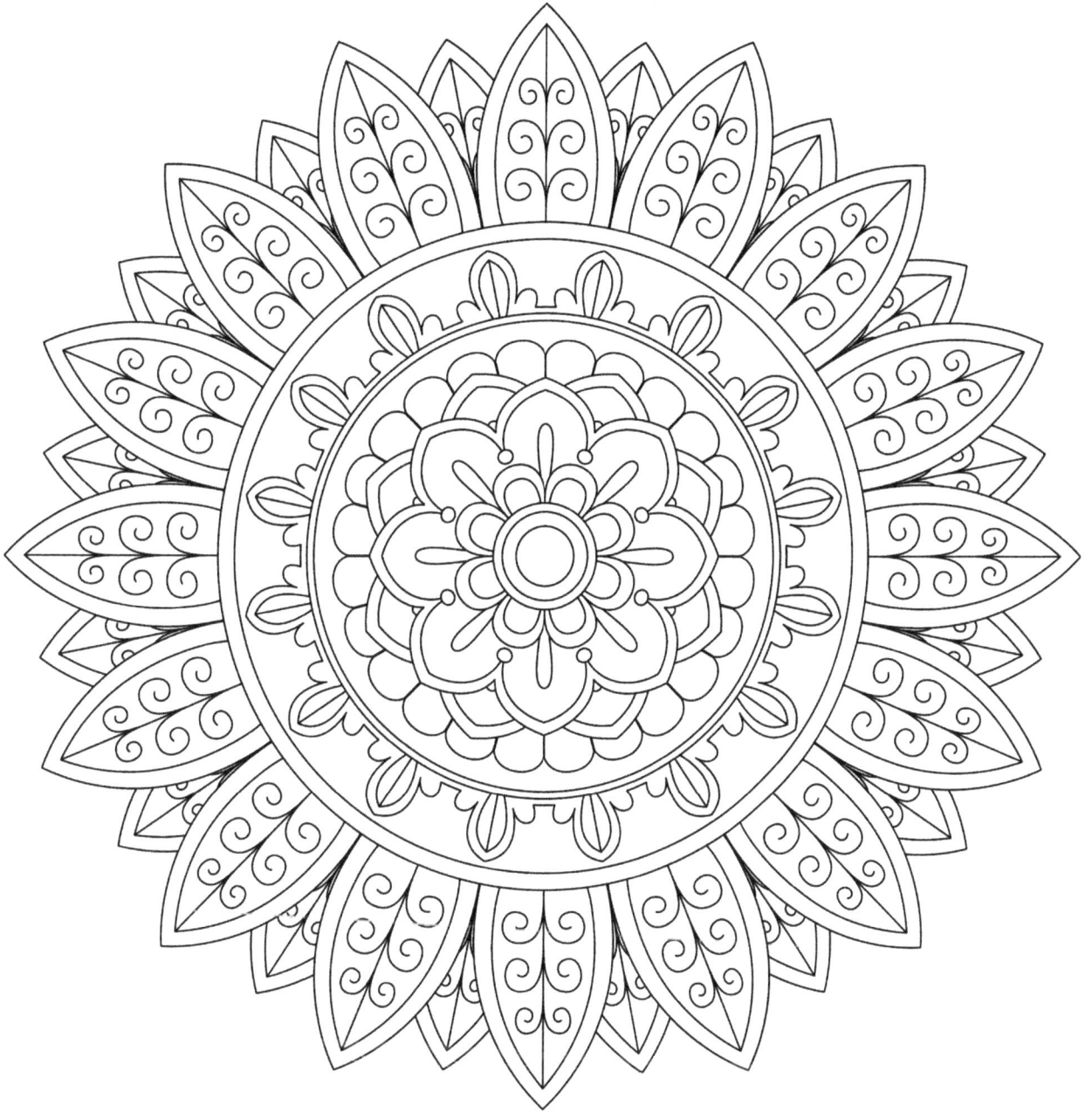

"Happiness is when what you think, what you say, and what you do are in harmony."

– Mahatma Gandhi

RELAX YOUR MIND ACTION PLAN

I recommend that you complete a weekly action plan as you continue your journey to realize your desired outcome and to *"Relax Your Mind."* An action plan will help to keep you focused on your desired outcome. It will also give you a record of your progress.

Consistent daily action will yield the best progress and results as you work towards your desired outcome. Your affirmation will help give you the focus and motivation. On the following pages, you will find an example weekly action plan and several blank weekly action plans to help get you started. Feel free to copy a blank one and use it for your weekly action steps.

The weekly action plan consists of the desired outcome, your affirmation, your practice action steps, and your experiences of your practices. Keep an open mind as you practice and be honest about your experiences so that you can better understand where you are along your journey. Remember that while practicing a little is better than not practicing at all, the more time you put into your practice, the better the results. And, remember to put a smile on your face and enjoy the journey as much as the destination.

Example Weekly Action Plan

Weekly Action Plan

Start Date: 8/17/00

Desired Outcome:

Calm at work while giving a presentation.

Affirmation:

I am calm as I give a clear and effective presentation at work.

Day	Action Steps (What action did I take?)	Experience (What did I feel/notice?)
Monday	I practiced silent witnessing for 30 minutes.	It was difficult to stay in the present moment.
Tuesday	I practiced abdominal breathing for 10 minutes.	I felt more relaxed as I continued to practice.
Wednesday	I took time to reflect on the fears causing my anxiety.	I was surprised by the fears that I identified.
Thursday	I practiced visualizing my desired outcome.	I was nervous at first, but then I calmed down.
Friday	I took a walk in the park in the present moment.	It was easier to stay in the present moment in nature.
Saturday	I practiced the relaxation meditation for 10 minutes	I felt calm and it was easier to visualize.
Sunday	I practiced the meditation for 7 minutes.	It was difficult to focus because of outside distractions.

Weekly Action Plan

Start Date: [ ]

Desired Outcome:

[ ]

Affirmation:

[ ]

Day	Action Steps (What action did I take?)	Experience (What did I feel/notice?)
Monday		
Tuesday		
Wednesday		
Thursday		
Friday		
Saturday		
Sunday		

Weekly Action Plan

Start Date: [ ]

Desired Outcome:

[ ]

Affirmation:

[ ]

Day	Action Steps (What action did I take?)	Experience (What did I feel/notice?)
Monday		
Tuesday		
Wednesday		
Thursday		
Friday		
Saturday		
Sunday		

Weekly Action Plan

Start Date: [   ]

Desired Outcome:

[   ]

Affirmation:

[   ]

Day	Action Steps (What action did I take?)	Experience (What did I feel/notice?)
Monday		
Tuesday		
Wednesday		
Thursday		
Friday		
Saturday		
Sunday		

Weekly Action Plan

Start Date: [ ]

Desired Outcome:

[ ]

Affirmation:

[ ]

Day	Action Steps (What action did I take?)	Experience (What did I feel/notice?)
Monday		
Tuesday		
Wednesday		
Thursday		
Friday		
Saturday		
Sunday		

NOTES

NOTES

ABOUT THE AUTHOR

Thomas Calabris has studied and practiced various forms of meditation and Qigong for almost thirty years. He studied meditation, Qigong, and Tai Chi from Grandmaster Robert Krueger. Most recently, he studied Inner Dan Arts Qigong (meditation and exercise) with Grandmaster Tianyou Hao, since January 2001. Thomas is a certified instructor of Inner Dan Arts Qigong. He also studied Qinway Qigong with Grandmaster Qinyin and Wisdom Healing Qigong with Master Mingtong Gu. He holds a Bachelor of Science Degree in Electrical Engineering and a Master of Science Degree in Biomedical Engineering. He currently develops software as a software engineer. He has also studied anatomy and physiology and various areas of natural health. He brings a unique perspective of science, tradition, and experience to his teachings.

Learn more about stress relief at:
http://www.EliminateStressNow.com

Learn more about Qigong at:
http://www.InnerVitalityQigong.com

OTHER BOOKS BY THE AUTHOR

Relax Your Mind: Simple Meditation Techniques to Relieve Stress and Quiet a Busy Mind

Learn more at: https://www.amazon.com/dp/173291060X

Healing Stress: Effective Solutions for Relieving Stress and Living a Stress-Free Life

Learn more at: https://www.amazon.com/dp/B07KVNXN14

The Color of Relaxation: Adult Coloring Book for Stress Relief and Relaxation

Learn more at: https://www.amazon.com/gp/product/1086248295

www.ingramcontent.com/pod-product-compliance
Lightning Source LLC
Chambersburg PA
CBHW081723270326
41933CB00017B/3278